CBD OIL FOR PAIN RELIEF

A comprehensive manual on managing chronic pain, anxiety, sleeplessness, and other conditions without experiencing psychoactive effects.

Dr. Amalie Kleist

1

Table of Contents

DISCLAIMER

This content is not meant to offer medical advice or replace advice or treatment from a personal physician. It is recommended that you get advice from your doctors or trained health specialists for any specific health inquiries you may have. Readers or followers of this instructional resource are responsible for any potential health effects.

INTRODUCTION

Dr. Amalie Kleist explores the remarkable impact of CBD oil on relieving chronic pain and improving quality of life in the book "CBD Oil for Pain Relief." This comprehensive guide provides a ray of hope for individuals struggling with painful conditions, supported by scientific research and real-life stories. Dr. Kleist delves into the scientific aspects of CBD's pain-relieving properties, explaining how it works and discussing dosage guidelines for various conditions. Learn about the way CBD interacts with the body's endocannabinoid system to regulate pain perception, offering a natural alternative to traditional pain medications without the usual side effects. This book offers more than just explanations; it acts as a guide to empowerment for those looking for alternatives to traditional pain management. Dr. Kleist provides valuable advice on choosing top-notch CBD products, overcoming legal obstacles, and integrating alternative treatments, empowering readers to manage their pain effectively. For those dealing with chronic pain or healthcare professionals looking for evidence-based solutions, "CBD Oil for Pain Relief" is a reliable guide to help you on your journey to wellness. Discover the countless people who have embraced CBD for its healing properties, and revitalize your well-being today. Discover the potential of nature's healing properties and say goodbye to discomfort with "CBD Oil for Pain Relief," the comprehensive healing manual by Dr. Amalie Kleist.

CHAPTER ONE

Introduction to CBD oil

What is CBD and CBD oil?

CBD is short for cannabidiol, a naturally occurring chemical included in the cannabis plant. Researchers have recognized it as one of more than 100 cannabinoids in cannabis. CBD is non-psychoactive, unlike tetrahydrocannabinol (THC), and does not induce the psychoactive effects commonly linked to marijuana consumption. CBD is becoming recognized for its potential medicinal advantages, such as alleviating pain, inflammation, anxiety, depression, seizures, and specific neurological conditions. It is commonly promoted and distributed in several formats, such as oils, capsules, lotions, gummies, and other edible products. Researchers are currently studying the medical uses of CBD. Some studies have shown encouraging results, but further research is required to comprehensively understand its effects and prospective applications. It is important to be aware that the legal status of CBD products varies depending on the location, and individuals should be cautious and seek advice from healthcare professionals before taking CBD products, particularly for medical reasons.

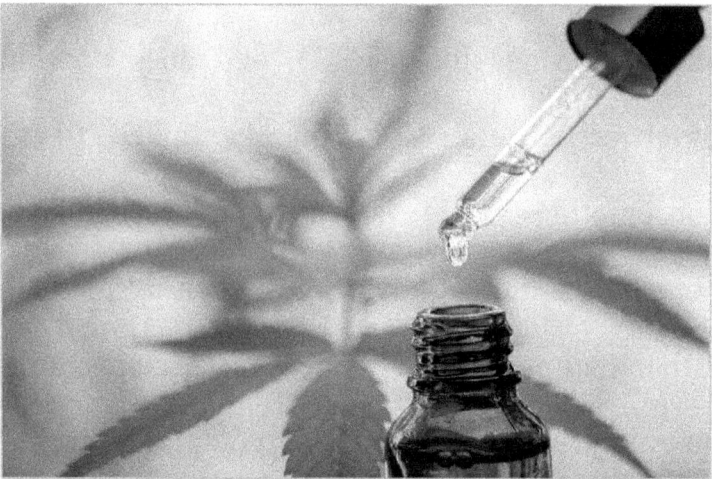

CBD oil is a concentrated liquid extract with elevated amounts of CBD content. Hemp plants, which have high CBD and low THC concentrations, usually yield the substance. Various sections of the hemp plant, like the flowers, leaves, and stalks, yield CBD oil. The solution is thinned by mixing it with a carrier oil like coconut oil or hemp seed oil to produce the end product.

Recently, CBD oil has become increasingly popular, attracting the interest of health enthusiasts, medical experts, and researchers. Extracted from the cannabis plant, CBD oil offers numerous potential benefits without causing the psychoactive effects often associated with tetrahydrocannabinol (THC). With the rising interest in natural medicines and alternative therapies, it is crucial to comprehend the basics of CBD oil.

Comprehending the
Endocannabinoid System

The endocannabinoid system (ECS) is a sophisticated biological system that is present in humans and other mammals. It is essential in controlling numerous physiological functions such as mood, memory, appetite, pain perception, immunological response, and inflammation. The ECS comprises three primary components:

1. **Endocannabinoids:** The body naturally creates endocannabinoids, which are endogenous lipid-based neurotransmitters. Anandamide (AEA) and 2-arachidonoylglycerol (2-AG) are the two main endocannabinoids. Cells produce the compounds in response to various physiological stimuli.

2. **Cannabinoid receptors:** There are two primary types of cannabinoid receptors, known as CB1 and CB2 receptors. CB1 receptors are mainly located in the central nervous system, specifically in the brain and spinal cord, whereas CB2 receptors are generally found in immune cells and peripheral organs. Endocannabinoids attach to these receptors to produce their effects.

3. **Enzymes:** Enzymes are in charge of both creating and breaking down endocannabinoids. Two crucial enzymes in this process are fatty acid amide hydrolase (FAAH), responsible for breaking down anandamide, and monoacylglycerol lipase (MAGL), responsible for breaking down 2-AG.

Neurotransmitters produced by the postsynaptic neuron interact with presynaptic receptors in the endocannabinoid system, operating through retrograde signaling. This process regulates neurotransmitter release and maintains homeostasis in the body. The Endocannabinoid System (ECS) has attracted considerable attention because of its role in several physiological and pathological states. It is involved in regulating pain, mood disorders, neurodegenerative illnesses, inflammation, metabolic problems, and other conditions. Therefore, the ECS modulation is being targeted for therapeutic interventions utilizing cannabinoids from cannabis plants (including THC and CBD) and synthetic cannabinoids to treat different medical ailments.

CHAPTER TWO

The benefits of CBD oil

Research on the potential benefits of CBD oil is in its initial phases, but early studies and anecdotal data indicate a broad spectrum of therapeutic uses.

Commonly cited benefits linked to CBD oil include:

- **Pain Relief:** CBD has analgesic characteristics that make it a viable alternative for addressing chronic pain diseases like arthritis, multiple sclerosis, and neuropathic pain.

- **Anxiety and Stress Reduction:** Users often find that CBD oil can ease symptoms of anxiety, stress, and depression. CBD influences serotonin receptors in the brain, potentially leading to its anxiety-reducing benefits.

- **Neuroprotective Properties:** CBD has been found to possess neuroprotective qualities, which could be advantageous for people suffering from neurodegenerative conditions including Alzheimer's and Parkinson's disease.

- **Anti-inflammatory Properties:** Prolonged inflammation is associated with several health issues, such as autoimmune diseases and heart ailments. The anti-inflammatory qualities of CBD may aid in reducing inflammation and enhancing overall health.

- **Sleep Improvement:** CBD oil has shown potential as a sleep aid, with numerous users reporting improved sleep quality and duration following the use of CBD supplements.

Uses of CBD oil

Uses of CBD Oil CBD oil has versatile applications for addressing diverse health issues and enhancing general well-being. Common applications of CBD oil include:

- **Pain Management:** To manage pain, CBD oil can be directly applied to aching muscles or joints for targeted pain relief. Orally administering it can also treat systemic pain and inflammation.

- **Epilepsy Treatment:** The U.S. Food and Drug Administration (FDA) has approved Epidiolex, a prescription CBD medicine, for treating rare types of epilepsy, such as Dravet syndrome and Lennox-Gastaut syndrome.

- **Anxiety and Stress Relief:** CBD oil can promote relaxation and alleviate anxiety and stress. One can consume it as tinctures, pills, or foods to manage anxiety.

- **Skin Care:** CBD-infused topicals like creams, lotions, and balms are becoming popular for their ability to treat skin disorders such as acne, eczema, and psoriasis.

- **Overall Wellbeing:** Many people incorporate CBD oil into their daily wellness regimen to support overall well-being, aiming to achieve balance and preserve optimal health.

Safety Measures

It is crucial to be mindful of certain safety measures when using CBD oil, as it is typically deemed safe for the majority of individuals

✓ **Quality and Purity:** Selecting premium CBD products from trustworthy suppliers is crucial to guaranteeing purity and effectiveness. Seek out products that have undergone third-party testing to ensure quality and safety.

✓ **Drug Interactions:** CBD can interact with specific pharmaceuticals such as blood thinners, antidepressants, and antiepileptic treatments. Prior to utilizing CBD oil, seek advice from your healthcare professional if you are using prescription drugs.

✓ **Side Effects:** Occasionally, individuals may encounter side effects like xerostomia, vertigo, queasiness, and changes in appetite while using CBD oil. Begin with a small dosage and observe your body's reaction to reduce the chances of negative outcomes.

✓ **Authorized Consideration:** Hemp-derived CBD oil is authorized in many regions; however, cannabis-derived CBD products may face more stringent regulations. Before purchasing or using

CBD oil, familiarize yourself with the laws and regulations governing CBD in your area before purchasing or using CBD oil.

As the study of CBD oil's therapeutic potential continues to grow, we can expect to learn more about how it works and what kinds of treatments it can help with. Ongoing clinical trials are investigating the efficacy of CBD for several medical diseases, showing encouraging outcomes in pain relief, anxiety treatment, and epilepsy control. CBD oil has potential in other domains beyond medicinal use, such as skincare, sports rehabilitation, and pet health. With increasing consumer interest in natural medicines and holistic wellness, CBD oil is expected to continue to have a significant presence in the health and wellness sector.

CHAPTER THREE

CBD Products

CBD products are available in a variety of forms, each designed to cater to diverse interests, lifestyles, and ingestion techniques. Having knowledge of the many categories of CBD products can assist individuals in selecting the most suitable solution for their needs.

There are several popular varieties of CBD products:

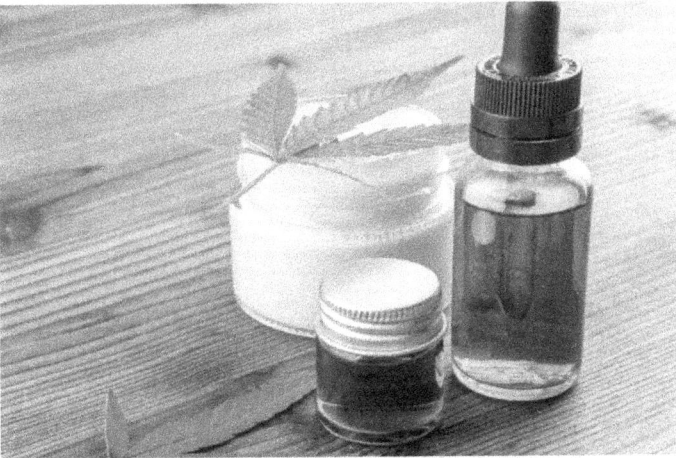

➢ **CBD Oil or Tinctures:** CBD oil or tinctures are a highly popular and diverse type of CBD product. They usually come in small containers with a dropper for convenient dosing. The sublingual method allows users to administer a small amount of CBD oil beneath their tongue for rapid absorption into the circulation. One can ingest CBD oil orally by adding it to meals or beverages.

➢ **CBD Edibles:** These are food products infused with CBD oil, such as gummies, chocolates, candies, and baked goods. Edibles provide a delicious and pleasant way to include CBD in one's everyday regimen. They are available in a variety of tastes and compositions, which makes them attractive to a wide range of people.

➢ **CBD Topicals:** CBD topicals provide targeted relief for pain, inflammation, and skin issues when applied directly to the skin. Typical CBD topicals consist of creams, lotions, balms, salves, and patches. Topicals provide precise alleviation by being absorbed transdermally and targeting specific regions of discomfort.

➢ **CBD Beverages:** CBD beverages, such as teas, coffees, waters, and sodas infused with CBD, are becoming increasingly popular as an alternate method of CBD consumption. These drinks provide a quick and pleasant way to stay hydrated while gaining the potential advantages of CBD.

➢ **CBD Vapes or Vape Oils:** CBD vape oils, or e-liquids, are specifically formulated for vaporizers or electronic cigarettes. Vaping enables CBD to be quickly absorbed into the circulation through the lungs, resulting in rapid symptom relief. When vaping, it is important to be cautious because the long-term consequences of inhaling CBD vape oil are currently under investigation.

➢ **Full-spectrum CBD Products:** Full-spectrum CBD products include a variety of cannabinoids, terpenes, and other helpful chemicals from the cannabis plant. These products utilize the combined effects of many plant components, referred to as the "entourage effect," to potentially boost the medicinal benefits of CBD.

➢ **CBD Isolate:** CBD isolate is the most refined form of CBD, usually found in crystalline powder or slab form. It exclusively includes CBD and lacks additional cannabinoids, terpenes, or plant components. You can include CBD isolate in foods, drinks, or homemade items to provide a personalized dosage.

➢ **CBD capsules or tablets:** CBD capsules or tablets provide an easy and inconspicuous method of ingesting CBD. Every capsule contains a specific quantity of CBD oil, simplifying dosage monitoring. Individuals who like a familiar and direct method of supplementing generally prefer capsules.

➤ **Broad-spectrum CBD Products:** Broad-spectrum CBD products include several cannabinoids and terpenes from the cannabis plant, except THC. They provide the advantages of the entourage effect while avoiding the potential for psychoactive effects associated with THC.

➤ **CBD for Pets:** CBD products designed for pets, like dogs and cats, come in different forms, like oils, snacks, and capsules. These items promote pet health by addressing concerns such as anxiety, pain, inflammation, and mobility problems.

When choosing a CBD product, it is crucial to investigate issues including preferred dosage, intake method, bioavailability, and personal preferences. Always buy

CBD products from trustworthy manufacturers that follow quality and safety requirements. Consult a healthcare practitioner before adding CBD to your wellness routine, especially if you have underlying health issues or are on drugs.

Common side effects associated with CBD oil products

Although CBD oil is typically harmless, it may induce negative effects in certain individuals. Typical adverse effects of taking CBD oil products may include:

- ✓ **Xerostomia:** CBD can reduce saliva production, causing dry mouth. Drinking water to hydrate yourself can help to reduce this sensation.

- ✓ **Vertigo:** Some individuals could feel drowsy or fatigued after consuming CBD oil, particularly in higher amounts. Avoid operating heavy machinery or driving a car until you comprehend the effects of CBD on your body.

✓ **Changes in appetite:** CBD can impact appetite, leading to either increased or decreased hunger in certain people. This effect is usually slight and transient.

✓ **Digestive issues:** CBD oil can lead to digestive problems, including diarrhea or nausea, in certain individuals, especially when consumed in large amounts.

✓ **Mood shifts:** Some people may notice mood shifts or heightened anxiety when initiating a new CBD routine or consuming high amounts, despite CBD being commonly used to reduce symptoms of anxiety and depression.

✓ **Drug interactions:** CBD can interact with specific drugs, potentially altering their efficacy.

Consulting a healthcare expert before using CBD oil is crucial, especially if you are on other medications or have underlying health concerns.

✓ **Liver enzyme elevation:** CBD oil can lead to higher liver enzyme levels, indicating potential liver inflammation or injury. Healthcare providers should closely monitor this uncommon side effect, especially in individuals with pre-existing liver disorders.

Begin with a small amount of CBD oil and slowly raise the dosage as necessary, while observing for any negative responses. Opting for premium CBD products from reputable manufacturers and seeking advice from a healthcare professional will reduce the likelihood of negative effects and ensure safe consumption.

CHAPTER FOUR

How is CBD oil extracted?

The hemp plant, a variant of the Cannabis sativa species, produces CBD oil from its flowers, leaves, and stalks. Each extraction technique for CBD oil has its own advantages and disadvantages. Here are a few prevalent techniques:

1. **CO2 Extraction**: This technique uses carbon dioxide (CO_2) under high pressure and low temperatures to separate, protect, and uphold the quality of the CBD oil. Although CO_2 extraction is a highly effective and environmentally friendly process, it requires expensive machinery.

2. **Steam distillation:** Steam distillation vaporizes the CBD oil by sending steam through the hemp plant

material. Condensing the vapor into liquid form isolates the CBD oil from the plant material. Due to its lower efficiency and potential degradation of heat-sensitive components, CBD extraction does not frequently utilize this approach.

3. **Solvent Extraction:** Solvent extraction utilizes solvents such as ethanol, butane, propane, or isopropyl alcohol to extract CBD from plant material. The solvent extracts the cannabinoids and other chemicals from the plant material. Evaporating the solvent after extraction results in the CBD oil. This process is more cost-effective than CO_2 extraction, but if not adequately removed, it could result in residual solvents in the end product.

4. **Extraction of hydrocarbons:** Hydrocarbon extraction uses hydrocarbons such as butane, propane, or hexane to extract CBD oil from plant

material. This process, like solvent extraction, can be quite effective but necessitates meticulous purging to eliminate any remaining hydrocarbons from the end product. Extraction method, initial hemp material, post-extraction processing, and testing processes influence the quality and purity of CBD oil.

5. **Extraction of Olive Oil:** Olive oil extraction is a secure and uncomplicated process that entails heating the plant material with olive oil to extract the cannabinoids. This process is less efficient than CO_2 or solvent extraction and yields a less concentrated product, but it is appropriate for making CBD oil at home.

Consumers should choose CBD products that have undergone testing by independent laboratories to verify their strength and purity, guaranteeing a safe and efficient product.

How to choose a quality CBD oil

It might be challenging to select high-quality CBD oil due to the wide variety of products on the market. When choosing a premium CBD oil, it is important to consider these critical factors:

> **Hemp Origin:** Look for CBD oils derived from organic hemp plants grown in the United States or Europe. Hemp plants are bioaccumulators, which indicates that they have the ability to absorb compounds from their surroundings. Organic farming reduces the risk of exposure to pesticides, herbicides, and other toxic chemicals.

> **Extraction Method**: The CO2 extraction method is widely regarded as the most superior technique for extracting CBD oil. This technique utilizes high pressure and low temperatures with carbon

dioxide to extract, retain, and uphold the purity of the CBD oil, guaranteeing the absence of any detrimental solvents or compounds.

➤ **Manufacturer's transparency and reputation:** Opt for CBD oil from companies that openly disclose their source, extraction techniques, and testing protocols. Seek out organizations with a strong reputation and favorable client feedback. CBD concentration: When selecting a CBD oil, it is crucial to choose a product with a concentration that aligns with your requirements and preferred dosage.

➤ **Full-Spectrum, Broad-Spectrum, or Isolate:** Choose from a full-spectrum, broad-spectrum, or CBD isolate product. Full-spectrum CBD includes all the naturally existing chemicals in the hemp plant, including minimal levels of THC (tetrahydrocannabinol). Broad-spectrum CBD includes several cannabinoids and terpenes, except THC. CBD isolate is CBD in its pure form, without any additional cannabinoids or terpenes.

➢ **Third-party Testing:** Reputable CBD companies provide third-party lab testing results. The tests confirm the effectiveness and cleanliness of the CBD oil, ensuring it has the stated CBD quantity and is uncontaminated by heavy metals, pesticides, or residual solvents.

➢ **Price:** Although not the only thing to consider, premium CBD oil usually has a higher price because of the quality of the components and extraction techniques employed. Exercise caution when considering products that are substantially less expensive than those available, as they can be of worse quality.

➢ **Customer reviews and suggestions:** Consult

customer reviews and solicit suggestions from acquaintances, relatives, or healthcare experts familiar with CBD oil. Their insights can assist you in making a well-informed selection.

By taking these variables into account, you can choose a premium CBD oil that meets your needs and delivers the intended therapeutic benefits.

CHAPTER FIVE

How to use CBD oil

To use CBD oil safely and effectively, it is important to follow specific protocols to determine the correct dosage. Here is a guide on how to use CBD oil:

✓ *Select the appropriate product*: CBD oil is available in different forms, including tinctures, capsules, edibles, topicals, and vape oils. Select a product that aligns with your interests and requirements.

✓ *Consult with a healthcare practitioner*: Prior to initiating CBD oil use, particularly if you have preexisting health concerns or are on medication, seek advice from a healthcare practitioner. They can provide tailored advice based on your health condition.

✓ *Begin with a Low Dosage*: Start with a small amount of CBD oil and then raise it until you determine the ideal dosage for your requirements. Initiating at a modest dose allows you to assess your body's reaction and reduces the risk of negative effects.

✓ *Follow the instructions:* Always adhere to the manufacturer's guidelines and the recommended dosage stated on the product label. Adhere to the requirements for safe and efficient use.

✓ *Sublingual Administration (Tinctures):*

- Carefully shake the bottle before using it to ensure the CBD extract is properly mixed.

- Administer the recommended dosage of CBD oil by placing the dropper underneath your tongue.

- Keep the oil beneath your tongue for 30–60 seconds

before swallowing to enhance absorption through the blood vessels under the tongue.

✓ *Taking CBD oil in the form of capsules or edibles:*

- Ingest capsules or eat CBD-infused edibles like you would any other dietary supplement or food product.

- Make sure you are aware of the amount and allow your body enough time to absorb the CBD.

✓ *Topical Use:*

- Administer CBD topicals directly to the skin in order to treat certain areas of pain or swelling.

- Massage the skin until it absorbs the topical product completely.

✓ *CBD oil vaping:*

- Utilize a vaporizer specifically created for CBD vape oil.

- Adhere to the manufacturer's guidelines while filling the vaporizer with CBD oil.

- Breathe in the vapor gradually and consistently.

✓ *Monitor the effects and adjust the dosage accordingly:* Observe your body's reactions to CBD oil. To obtain the desired benefits, adjust the dosage or frequency of use as necessary.

✓ *Be consistent:* Consistency is crucial while utilizing CBD oil. Integrate it into your daily routine for the best long-term results.

✓ *Proper Storage:* Keep your CBD oil in a cool, dry location shielded from direct sunlight to preserve its strength and freshness.

✓ *Monitor for Adverse Reactions:* Although CBD is usually well-tolerated, certain individuals may encounter side effects such as xerostomia, sleepiness, diarrhea, or alterations in appetite. If you encounter any bad reactions, discontinue use and consult with a healthcare practitioner.

By adhering to these instructions, you can safely and efficiently utilize CBD oil to potentially manage different health issues and enhance general wellness.

Dosage guidelines for CBD oil usage

The recommended dosage of CBD oil can differ based on variables like body weight, personal tolerance, CBD concentration, condition severity, and delivery route. Begin with a small dosage and incrementally raise it until you reach the most effective dose for your requirements. Here are some standard dose recommendations:

- **START LOW**

Begin treatment with a low dose, usually ranging from 5–10 mg of CBD per day, particularly if you are inexperienced with CBD oil. Initiating at a modest dose enables you to assess your body's reaction and reduce the risk of negative effects.

- **INCREASE GRADUALLY**

Progressively increase the dosage by 5–10 mg every few days if the intended benefits are not achieved until the desired outcomes are obtained.

- **TAKE INTO CONSIDERATION BODY WEIGHT**

Typically, people with a higher body weight may need higher dosages of CBD than those with a lower body weight.

- **ADHERE TO PRODUCT RECOMMENDATIONS**

Consult the manufacturer's dosing instructions on the product label. CBD oil products usually specify the CBD concentration per serving.

- **CONCENTRATION**

Consider the product's CBD concentration. If you have a tincture with 1000 mg of CBD in a 30 mL bottle, each mL will contain approximately 33 mg of CBD.

- **TALK TO A MEDICAL PROFESSIONAL**

Seek advice from a healthcare expert if you are uncertain about the correct dosage, have underlying health issues, or are on medication before using CBD oil. They can offer tailored guidance according to your specific situation.

- **KEEP AN EYE OUT FOR REACTIONS**

Monitor your body's reaction to CBD oil. If you encounter any negative reactions or pain, you should either change the dosage or stop using the product.

- **BE CONSISTENT**

Consistency in dose is crucial for maximizing the effectiveness of CBD oil. Incorporate it into your daily routine and follow a consistent dosage plan.

- **TAKE INTO ACCOUNT THE METHOD OF ADMINISTRATION**

The way a substance is administered might impact the required dosage and the time it takes for effects to begin. Sublingual administration, such as placing the substance under the tongue, may produce quicker results than consuming CBD oil in pill or edible form.

- **EXERCISE PATIENCE**

It may take time to discover the optimal dosage that suits you. Exercise patience and allow your body sufficient time to adapt and react to the CBD oil.

Keep in mind that the effects of CBD oil might differ from person to person, meaning what is effective for one individual may not be effective for another. It is crucial to pay attention to your body and modify the dosage as needed to get the desired results while reducing the risk of unwanted effects.

Methods of consuming CBD oil:

Benefits and Drawbacks

Of course! Let's examine the various ways of ingesting CBD oil, along with their benefits and drawbacks.

INGESTION (CAPSULES, EDIBLES)

Benefits:

- Easy dosing: capsules and edibles provide predetermined amounts, making administration easy.

- No flavor: capsules and snacks conceal the flavor of CBD oil.

- Prolonged effects: CBD has prolonged effects due to its gradual release as it traverses the digestive system.

Drawbacks:

- Slow onset: CBD's effects are slower when ingested as it must travel through the digestive system, in contrast to sublingual delivery.

- Variable absorption: CBD's absorption can vary depending on the processes of digestion and metabolism, resulting in lower bioavailability when ingested.

CBD CONCENTRATES

Benefits:

- High effectiveness: CBD concentrates have elevated amounts of CBD, providing strong benefits.

- Flexibility: Concentrates offer flexibility as they can be ingested through dabbing, vaping, or by adding them to food or beverages.

Drawbacks:

- Specialized equipment is required for dabbing and

vaping CBD concentrates.

- Potency issue: Concentrates with high potency levels could be too intense for inexperienced users.

- Cost: CBD concentrates may have a higher price point compared to other types of CBD products.

TOPICAL ADMINISTRATION

Benefits:

- Targeted relief: Topical treatments are well-suited for specific areas of discomfort, inflammation, and skin issues.

- Non-psychoactive: CBD topicals do not reach the bloodstream, so they do not induce psychoactive effects.

- Simple to use: Applying topicals to the affected area is easy and immediate.

Drawbacks:

- Restricted systemic effect: Topical treatments offer relief in a specific area and may not affect the entire system.

- Skin irritation risk: Certain individuals may develop skin irritation or allergic reactions to topical products.

SUBLINGUAL TINCTURE ADMINISTRATION

Benefits:

- Rapid absorption: CBD quickly enters the bloodstream through the sublingual blood vessels.

- Accurate dosage management: Tinctures typically include droppers for precise measurement.

- Carrying tinctures is convenient and drinking them can be done discreetly.

Drawbacks:

- Some individuals may perceive the flavor of CBD

oil as irritating.

- Not suitable for individuals who have trouble retaining liquids beneath their tongue.

VAPING

Benefits:

- Quick absorption: CBD rapidly enters the bloodstream via the lungs, resulting in immediate benefits.

- Increased bioavailability: Due to its high bioavailability, vaping increases CBD absorption into the circulation more efficiently.

- Adjustable dosing: Users have the ability to customize the dosage by changing the amount of puffs.

Drawbacks:

- Health concerns: Risks to health arise from an

incomplete understanding of the long-term effects of vaping and the potential dangers involved with inhalation of vaporized drugs.

- Essential equipment: Vaping requires specialized tools such as vaporizers or vape pens.

- Lung irritation: Vaping may cause lung inflammation or have negative effects on the respiratory system in some people.

CBD FLOWER SMOKING

Benefits:

- Quick-acting: Smoking CBD flowers delivers effects rapidly, similar to vaping.

- Natural product: CBD flower is a natural and minimally processed type of CBD.

- Adjustable dosing: Users can customize the dosage by regulating the quantity of smoked flower.

Drawbacks:

- Health hazards: Inhaling any drug through smoking can endanger respiratory health.

- Legal issue: The legality of smoking a CBD flower depends on the jurisdiction.

- Psychoactive effects: This may occur with certain CBD flower strains due to the presence of tiny quantities of THC.

When selecting a way to consume CBD oil, it is crucial to take into account elements like start time, duration of effects, bioavailability, convenience, personal preferences, and potential health hazards. It is recommended to begin with a small dose of CBD oil and slowly raise it as necessary while observing how your body reacts. Consulting a healthcare practitioner can help determine the most appropriate manner of intake tailored to individual requirements and health concerns. Topical administration:

CHAPTER 6

Integrating CBD oil into daily routines

CBD, or cannabidiol, has garnered interest in the fitness and wellness world for its potential advantages in aiding recovery and promoting general well-being.

Here is how CBD can be included in workout regimens and recovery:

PAIN RELIEF AND INFLAMMATION REDUCTION

CBD has anti-inflammatory properties that can help to alleviate muscular soreness and inflammation following vigorous exercise or physical activity. This could help expedite recovery and alleviate discomfort linked to muscular strains or injuries.

ENHANCED SLEEP QUALITY

Quality sleep is crucial for muscle healing and overall health. CBD can enhance sleep quality by alleviating anxiety and inducing relaxation, resulting in improved restorative sleep patterns.

SEVERAL ADMINISTRATION METHODS

CBD is available in several administration methods, including oils, capsules, topical creams, and edibles, giving users the flexibility to select the approach that suits their preferences and requirements. Topical CBD treatments can directly alleviate pain in specific muscles, while oral CBD medications can provide widespread effects.

ANXIETY AND STRESS REDUCTION

Engaging in high-intensity workouts and hard training may raise stress levels. CBD has demonstrated anxiolytic effects, which could assist individuals in coping with stress and anxiety related to rigorous physical training.

IMPROVED FOCUS AND CONCENTRATION

Certain individuals have noted that CBD can enhance focus and concentration, potentially aiding in workouts or training.

A SUBSTITUTE FOR NSAIDS

Numerous athletes and fitness enthusiasts depend on nonsteroidal anti-inflammatory drugs (NSAIDs) for pain management, but these treatments can lead to adverse effects when used over an extended period of time. CBD is a natural option for controlling pain and inflammation without the possible dangers linked to NSAIDs.

PERSONALIZED DOSAGE

Determining the correct amount of CBD is essential for attaining the best outcomes. Start with a small dosage and gradually increase it until you achieve the desired benefits. It is crucial to pay attention to your body's signals and modify the dosage accordingly.

CONSULT WITH AN ANXIETY HEALTHCARE EXPERT

Consult a healthcare expert before incorporating CBD into your exercise and recuperation regimen, especially if you have underlying health issues or are on medication, to confirm its safety and suitability for you.

ANXIETY PERFORMANCE IS ALLEVIATED

CBD can alleviate performance anxiety in athletes and individuals, leading to improved mental clarity and reduced nervousness, ultimately enhancing performance in exercises or contests.

Although numerous individuals share favorable encounters with CBD for physical fitness and recuperation, individual reactions can differ. Using premium CBD products from trustworthy sources is crucial, and it's essential to consider any possible conflicts with prescriptions or current health issues.

Cooking with CBD oil

Using CBD oil in cooking may be an enjoyable and innovative way to incorporate the potential benefits of CBD into your meals.

Nevertheless, it is crucial to remember a few key points to maximize the benefits of your CBD-infused meals:

- Opt for premium CBD oil

Go for premium CBD oil tailored for culinary purposes to ensure quality. Seek out items identified as "food-grade" or "culinary CBD oil" to guarantee their safety and quality.

- Determine Dosage

Establish the correct amount of CBD oil needed for your recipe. Begin with a modest quantity and incrementally raise it as necessary, while adhering to the suggested serving size for the particular CBD oil you have.

- Avoid high temperatures

CBD oil is heat-sensitive and can lose its effectiveness if exposed to high temperatures for a prolonged period of time. To maintain the beneficial qualities of CBD, avoid using high heat when cooking and opt for low-heat methods such as sautéing or baking at lower temperatures.

- Put CBD oil at the right time

Integrate CBD oil into your dishes at the end of the cooking process, after removing the dish from the heat, to minimize the risk of CBD degradation due to heat exposure.

- Incorporating flavors

CBD oil possesses a unique earthy taste that might not suit all palates. Pair it with flavors like citrus, herbs, spices, or sweets to improve the taste of your dishes and cover up any bitterness from the CBD oil.

- Keep flavors in check

Consider the overall flavor profile of your food and adjust the amount of CBD oil to ensure it complements the other ingredients without being too strong.

- Explore Various Recipes

Be innovative and try out numerous recipes to discover pleasant ways to include CBD oil in your preferred cuisine. The options are limitless, ranging from salad dressings and sauces to baked items and beverages.

- Proper Storage

Keep your CBD oil in a cool, dark location, shielded from direct sunlight and heat, to preserve its freshness and effectiveness.

- Monitor serving sizes

Track the quantity of CBD oil used in each recipe, and be aware of the combined impact if you consume numerous servings in a day. By adhering to these guidelines, you can successfully integrate CBD oil into your culinary creations and savor the potential advantages of CBD in a range of delectable meals.

CHAPTER 7

Frequently Asked Questions (FAQs)

Below are some frequently asked questions (FAQs) about CBD (cannabidiol), along with their responses:

1. *What is CBD?*

CBD, or cannabidiol, is an inherent chemical present in the cannabis plant. It is among more than 100 cannabinoids found in cannabis.

2. *What key distinctions exist between THC and CBD?*

CBD and THC differ mainly in their psychoactive effects. THC is psychoactive and can change perception, mood, and cognitive functioning, while CBD is non-intoxicating. Many areas allow CBD, while many countries still prohibit THC.

3. *Does CBD cause psychoactive effects?*

CBD does not produce the intoxicating effects associated with marijuana. THC, or tetrahydrocannabinol, is the chemical component that causes the psychoactive effects commonly linked to cannabis, not CBD. CBD products may include small quantities of THC, usually insufficient to induce intoxication.

4. What are the possible medicinal advantages of CBD and THC?

Researchers have studied the potential medicinal benefits of both CBD and THC. CBD is commonly used for its purported benefits in relieving pain, anxiety, sadness, seizures, inflammation, and various other issues. THC may possess medicinal effects such as pain alleviation, nausea reduction, hunger stimulation, and muscle relaxation.

5. What are the potential health benefits of CBD?

Research has explored the possible therapeutic benefits

of CBD, such as alleviating pain, anxiety, depression, sleeplessness, seizures, and inflammation. Further research is required to comprehensively grasp its effectiveness and possible applications.

6. Is CBD legal?

CBD's legality is contingent on its source and the jurisdiction's legislation. Various areas of the United States federally permit CBD derived from hemp with less than 0.3% THC. Laws concerning CBD can differ significantly across various countries or states.

7. What is the proper method for consuming CBD?

CBD products are available in several forms, such as oils, tinctures, capsules, edibles, topicals, and vape goods. The technique of ingestion varies depending on the individual choice and the intended outcomes. Adhering to the manufacturer's recommended dose guidelines is crucial.

8. Do CBD products have any adverse effects?

Although CBD is often safe for the majority of individuals, possible side effects might include tiredness, xerostomia, diarrhea, changes in appetite, and interactions with specific drugs. Before consuming CBD, consult a healthcare expert, especially if you have any preexisting health concerns or are on medication.

9. *How long does it take for CBD to start working?*

Factors such as administration method, dosage, metabolism, and the specific condition being treated can influence the timing and duration of CBD effects. The effects of vaping CBD can be experienced within minutes, whereas the effects of consuming CBD edibles or capsules may take up to an hour or more to be felt.

10. *Is it safe to administer CBD to my pets?*

Pet owners utilize CBD products for their pets to alleviate pain, anxiety, and other ailments. It is crucial to utilize CBD products designed for pets and to seek advice from a veterinarian before administering CBD to your pet to guarantee safety and the correct dosage.

11. *Is it permissible to travel with CBD?*

When traveling, transporting CBD can be difficult because of inconsistent rules. Research and adhere to the laws of the jurisdiction you are traveling to and from, as well as the transportation method you are utilizing. Transporting CBD products over state or international boundaries may be illegal in some situations.

These FAQs provide fundamental information about CBD, but it is critical to conduct more research or seek advice from a healthcare expert for tailored counsel and information.

Future of CBD research and regulations

- **Expanding Research:** The enthusiasm for CBD research was rapidly increasing. Scientists were investigating its possible therapeutic uses for illnesses like anxiety, chronic pain, epilepsy, and others. As rescarch advances, scientists anticipate gaining more knowledge about the effectiveness and safety of CBD.

- **Clinical trials:** recognizing the necessity for stronger scientific research to verify the medicinal benefits linked to CBD. Researchers anticipated that advancements in research would provide additional clinical trials to scientifically validate the effectiveness and safety of CBD for various medical conditions.

- **Quality and safety standards:** Efforts were made to create quality and safety standards for CBD products.

Regulators and industry stakeholders were collaborating to set standards for CBD products to guarantee consumer safety and proper labeling, addressing issues including product uniformity, contaminants, and misleading labels.

- **Consumer literacy:** As CBD products gained popularity, there was an increased need for consumer education. It was essential to offer precise details about CBD, including its advantages, correct usage, and hazards, to help people make well-informed decisions.

- **Emerging Applications:** In addition to established therapeutic purposes, there was a curiosity about investigating novel uses of CBD, such as in skincare, cosmetics, and wellness items. Advancements in research and innovation in these fields could lead to an expansion of CBD products and markets.

- **International Harmonization:** Attempts were underway to standardize CBD legislation globally. This was crucial for enhancing international trade, guaranteeing product quality and safety, and advocating for uniform regulatory methods worldwide.

- **Regulatory Clarity:** The CBD regulatory framework was developing. Many jurisdictions were developing or updating regulations for the manufacturing, sale, and marketing of CBD products. This regulatory environment will continue to influence the CBD sector and consumers' ability to purchase CBD products.

By 2024, it is probable that these trends will continue to influence the CBD research and regulation environment. Specific advancements may differ based on variations in legislation, scientific findings, and industry trends across different locations. It is critical to stay abreast of the most recent research discoveries and regulatory changes.

ACKNOWLEDGEMENTS

All glory belongs to God. I'd also want to thank my wonderful family, partner, fans, readers, friends, and customers for their constant support and words of encouragement.